Nutrisystem

A Beginner's 20-Minute Overview, Review, and
Analysis of the Diet Plan

Disclaimer

By reading this disclaimer, you are accepting the terms of the disclaimer in full. If you disagree with this disclaimer, please do not read the guide. The content in this guide is provided for informational and educational purposes only.

This guide is not intended to be a substitute for the original work of this diet plan. At most, this guide is intended to be a beginner's supplement to the original work for this diet plan and never act as a direct substitute. This guide is an overview, review, and commentary on the facts of that diet plan.

Always seek the advice of your physician or another qualified health provider with any issues or questions you might have regarding any sort of medical condition. Do not ever disregard any qualified professional medical advice or delay seeking that advice because of anything you have read in this guide.

Table of Contents

Introduction

What food comes to your mind when I say the word diet-food? I am sure that this word conjures images of nuts, oats, vegetables, and tasteless dishes. Perhaps it a heaping pile of dark veggies like spinach and kale.

On the other hand, what would you think of if I say these foods? Smores Pie. Buttermilk Waffles. Pepperoni Pizza Melt. Lasagna with Meat Sauce. Milk Chocolate Flavored Pretzels. I am sure that the words that popped up were delicious and unhealthy.

But what if I tell you that those are diet-food? Those dishes are a part of Nutrisystem's menu for their weight-loss program.

It may sound unusual at first, but having choices such as these is precisely why this service is so attractive to many of its users.

This brief guide aims to provide a high level beginner's overview of what the Nutrisystem diet is all about. The guide then goes into an analysis of the pros and cons of this diet program, and ultimately concludes with a recommendation.

In this diet plan review you will discover:
- What Nutrisystem is
- How it works
- My experience with the program
- The pros and cons
- What Nutrisystem plans are available
- What are its alternatives

Chapter 1: What is Nutrisystem?

Nutrisystem was founded in 1972 in Pennsylvania by entrepreneur Harold Katz. It was a commercial provider of weight loss products and services from the very beginning. In 1999 it moved to a direct-to-consumer business model, selling its products through the internet and call centers. In 2010 the company's mobile platform was launched.

Today its main product is a 4-week program that provides ready-made, pre-proportioned meals, and snacks that focus primarily on low caloric intake which will lead to weight loss. This program has been sponsored by numerous celebrities including Janet Jackson, Melissa Joan Hart, and Dan Marino.

Chapter 2: How Does it Work?

Nutrisystem, to put it simply, makes eating healthy food for weight loss convenient.

They prepare an easy program for its users to follow and, more importantly, provide easy to prep meals. And when they say easy, they do mean easy, as most of their items are ready to eat right out of the package or you simply need to reheat them. What you will be typically getting are 6 meals per day for 20 days (breakfast, lunch, dinner, 3x snacks). You will be consuming these during the weekdays while on the weekends you are free to eat what you want as long as you follow the guidelines placed in their program.

Each meal that you get are healthier versions of your favorite food. One of the hardest parts when it comes to dieting is the fact that most of them involve cutting out sugar, salt, and fat, which unfortunately leaves out a lot of our favorite food, especially processed ones. But as mentioned at the start of this review, the food you will be getting is food that you are familiar with.

However, Nutrisystem makes sure that their food still provides the right mix of nutrients, plenty of healthy and lean protein, high fiber, low-glycemic carbs, and no artificial sweeteners or flavors. You can have a hamburger without worrying about your health, or your belly when you eat the food they provide.

At its heart, the Nutrisystem diet place focuses on lowering its user's caloric intake. You will be eating around 1,200 to 1,500 calories per day. This is why it works so well in helping its customers lose weight. Also by eating every 2 to 3 hours, this helps you get full for a longer time.

This program will also come with a guidebook, helping you on those days that you have no prepared meals. It also works in conjunction with their free NuMi weight loss app which has fun challenges, prizes, tips, recipes, and more.

Chapter 3: My Experience With the Program

The moment I first heard about this program I was interested in trying it out. I have already tried different diets from the no carbs diet to the keto diet. The hardest thing about these diets is having to prepare the meals. When I heard that Nutrisystem was going to prepare most of my meals for me as well as provide me food that will not make me feel like a rabbit, I was in.

At the start of the program, I received two huge boxes, one of them containing pre-packed snacks and meals, the other containing frozen goods. I had to clean a lot of things out of my freezer, as I had not thought about the amount of food I was getting. But everything looked good and I could already feel the convenience oozing out of their product as each meal is packed individually and looks like something I would get out of the grocery.

In my first week, I had an easy time adjusting to the system. It was different though from what I was going to have in the next three weeks as I had to drink a protein shake as my first snake, which is provided in the box. I think even though I had fewer calories during this time than normal I still felt relatively full throughout the day. I never felt hungry at any point because of the amount, and quality, of the food I ate. However, after only one week I already lost 7 pounds. A lot of it was probably water weight but still, I barely felt I was on a diet.

Week two up to week four was also easy for me. I had gotten used to the program by then. On the weekends, even if I did not have prepared meals, it was quick for me to adjust my eating habits. I just had to focus on portion control and I was mindful of the caloric content of what I was eating. The best part was I was still able to go out with my friends without having to worry too much about which food to choose. I just picked what I wanted, divided it into a smaller portion with the remaining food set aside for my dog, and enjoyed the company of my friends. It was not as stressful as it was when I was trying out different diets as before, having the option to only pick a very limited amount of foods that I could eat.

PROS

Convenience – I cannot stress this enough, the Nutrisystem is convenient. I did not have to worry about prepping, cooking, and packing my meals as I did before. I mean even when I was eating normally I did so much work for my daily meals. By having my meals in a convenient package I was able to just grab them and stuff them in my bag to take them to work. (I had an insulated bag for the frozen items.) This to me alone is the biggest help that this system was able to give me.

Affordability - This was very affordable. The Nutrisystem meal plan starts at $8.57 a day. This gets you around 120 meals (20 days x 6 meals a day) and gives you guidelines on the days that you do not have a meal ready. Let me make their pricing a bit clear though just because I want my readers to have no illusion as to what they are going to be paying. First of all, it is a little bit more expensive for men. For the package that costs $8.57 a day, it costs $10 a day for men. Second, the daily rate posted on their site is for the 4-week fee divided into 28 days. You are not technically just paying for $8.57/$10 for one day's worth of meals. You are paying $12-$14 per daily meals. But even at that price, it is affordable as you are paying for the convenience and the prospective of weight loss.

Menu choices - Lastly, because this diet focuses on calorie-cutting, their food choices are outstanding. You will not be stuck with eating raw carrot sticks or some kind of flaxseed cereal mix. Let me give you an example of the things I could eat in one day.

Breakfast – Turkey sausage and egg muffin
First snack – White cheddar popcorn
Lunch – Meatball parmesan melt
Second snack – Chocolate pretzel bar
Dinner – Sausage pizza
Third snack – Carrot cake

Nothing in that list screams diet food. It is one of the things that I loved best when doing the Nutrisystem diet. It allowed me to enjoy a lot of foods that I enjoyed before while still helping me lose pounds. A word of warning though, the meal listed above contains three Nutrisystem snacks but usually for two of the snacks you will be forced to come up with your own.

As a bonus, the food that you receive will come with educational materials. While I am already familiar with a lot of the concepts discussed in those pamphlets, I can see how it would be really helpful for total beginners. While the biggest value you can get from doing the Nutrisystem plan is the actual meals, having the training to pick what things to buy in the grocery is an important skill to have. This will especially come in handy if you do choose to stop using Nutrisystem in the future.

CONS

It is hard to come up with cons for this program. I think the hardest part for me was that I had to do my food on the weekends. But at the same time, it also trained me to be more aware of what I am putting into my body so I did not mind as much.

Also since this diet is focused on counting calories it is hard to do heavy exercises. You can do light exercises, which they suggest that you do, but unless you want to feel weak, avoid planning physically intensive activities for the weeks you're doing this program.

Aside from those, there is not much else that is bad with this product. I do not want to sound like I am a sponsor for this product (I'm not) but it is a great one. It is convenient, affordable, and delicious. There's almost no reason not to get it if you do want to lose weight without stressing too much.

Chapter 4: How Their Plan Works

Their website URL is nutrisystem.com. If you click the large orange order button on the right, and select which plan you want to have. Nutrisystem offers a variety of plans, including ones that cater to people with diabetes or those with a vegetarian diet. For this review, though I will focus on their three main plans, Basic, Uniquely Yours, and Uniquely Yours Ultimate.

Before I point out the differences though I would like to go through some of the similarities. All plans have two choices when it comes to the menu. You can either choose to have Nutrisystem pick your meals for you (Chef's Choice), which consists of their best selling products, and would be a good way to get taste their dishes, or you choose which dishes you like. If you do opt for choosing the dishes be sure to check out the details of each dish. By clicking on a dish it will show you reviews left by customers on that particular dish, Q&As regarding the dish, ingredients, nutritional content, and preparation method.

Another similarity is that all of the plans will still require you to prepare your food once in a while. The guidebook included that I mentioned earlier will be helpful for this along with the Niu app as both have the grocery shopping guidelines listed as well as recipes to try. This happens because while the Nutrisystem pushes you to eat six times a day (breakfast, lunch, dinner, and three snack times) they only provide three main meals and one snack per day. Not to mention in two of the days you're left to your own devices.

One last similarity is that for men an additional snack will be given as men need more calories. This means that the price is a tad bit higher for men than women.

Basic plan

The basic plan costs $239.99 for four weeks ($8.57 per day) for women and $279.99 for four weeks ($10.00 per day) for men. The biggest difference between this plan and the others is that the menu choices for it are limited as frozen dishes are not included. This might be a huge drawback for some though as a lot of the more popular choices are frozen. However, the price is affordable for someone who wants to try out the service. And the food choices are still not bad. You have 20 choices for breakfast, 22 for lunch, 16 for dinner, and 33 for snack time. For breakfast, lunch, and dinner, you get to choose 22 dishes while for snack time you get to choose 37 snacks. Personally, while this is the most affordable choice of all three, the semi-limited options are the main reason why I did not pick this plan. However, if you just want to try out the system and not have to worry about cleaning your freezer to make way for frozen items, this would be a good choice for you.

Uniquely Yours plan

This was the plan that I got for myself. The plan costs $289.99 for four weeks ($10.36 per day) for women and $329.99 for four weeks ($11.79 per day) for men. According to the website, this is the most popular plan and it is easy to see why. For just $50 more you get access to a wider variety of dishes (I think the Turkey Sausage & Egg Muffin alone is worth it but that is just my opinion). This time you have 33 choices for breakfast, 39 for lunch, 31 for dinner, and 42 for snacks. The number of meals you order per meal is still the same though as you still get to order 22 dishes each for breakfast, lunch, and dinner, while you get to choose 37 snacks for snack time. I chose this one because a lot of the frozen items were really attractive to me.

Uniquely Yours Ultimate plan

This plan is mainly for those who want to do less cooking as it adds in more prepared food in the shipment. The plan costs $349.99 for four weeks ($12.50 per day) for women and $389.99 for four weeks ($13.93 per day) for men. As for the choices, the number remains the same with the Uniquely Yours plan, with 33 choices for breakfast, 39 for lunch, 31 for dinner, and 42 for snacks. However this time you get to order 28 meals for breakfast, lunch, and dinner, and 49 snacks for snack time. So for the extra $60 you get 6 days' worth of meals in this plan. I would pick this if I have work to do on the weekends as this would make it much easier for me. I think the additional meals that only costs $10 a day is a great deal.

Now as I mentioned earlier Nutrisystem also offers other plans other than the ones I listed above. I will give a quick run-through of each one.

Vegetarian plan - $289.99 for four weeks for women and $329.99 for four weeks for men. You have 28 choices for breakfast, 19 choices for lunch, 7 choices for dinner, and 41 choices for snacks. You then order 22 meals for breakfast, lunch, and dinner, and 37 snacks for snack time. This deal is the same as Uniquely Yours except that the meals have been filtered to only show the vegetarian dishes. As far as I can see there are no special vegetarian meals that are exclusive to this plan.

Diabetes plans – There are three diabetes plans and it is just the same as the regular one – Basic, Uniquely Yours, and Uniquely Yours Ultimate. Just as with the Vegetarian plan the prices are the same as the corresponding regular plans. The number of choices available was interesting as except for one or two dishes all the choices that are available for the regular plans are also available in these plans, without any changes as they were all diabetes-friendly in the first place. I think the biggest difference for this plan is that you get access to certified diabetes instructors. Also, you will not have a different meal plan for the first week, unlike the other plans.

Nutrisystem Your Way – This plan allows you to customize the number of Nutrisystem meals that you want to receive. For example, you can choose to order more meals for lunch and dinner than for breakfast as you think you have more time to prepare for it anyway. If more control over the number of Nutrisystem meals is more important for you then this would be a good choice for you.

So now that you have picked a plan, all you have to do is wait. Once it arrives here are some things that you will have to do.

1) Prepare your space

As I mentioned earlier you will be receiving a lot of food. If you chose the Basic plan this might not be that big of a deal but for the Uniquely Yours plan I ended up dumping everything I had in my freezer before receiving my Nutrisystem meals just to accommodate all the frozen items I received.

2) Organize everything

In the beginning, I had such a hard time going through my planned Nutrisystem meals until I realized that I should have already organized them by day right from the start. Do not do it as I did and just stash everything in one go at the beginning.

3) Read the guides in the boxes

Trust me on this. I know that our instinct with instructions is to usually set it aside but in this case, it would be good for you to get familiar with the principles of the Nutrisystem diet as well as how to create Flex meals – meals that you prepare on your own for the days that you have no Nutrisystem meals available.

4) Track your measurements

Make sure that you measure your weight and your waistline every single day. This helps you keep track of your weight loss and to be honest, it is quite encouraging to see your weight drop. I know it helped me continue this diet after seeing my weight drop in just a day or two.

Chapter 5: Alternatives to this Program

Medifast – There are numerous low-calorie meal providers in the market similar to Nutrisystem. One such program is Medifast. I have a friend who tried this out and after comparing notes it seems to be fairly similar although the target calories seem to be a bit lower for them. There are other diet meal companies out there as well such as HMR and Optifast with the major difference being the meals that they offer so you might want to check these out if you do want other options

Weight watchers- This is a different service from what Nutrisystem offers. Instead of providing meals, it offers guidance, coaching, and support. It is cheaper than Nutrisystem and in terms of weight loss, US News ranks it as number one in their weight loss diets. The hardest part here is that you will still have to make your meals however constant coaching would probably help encourage you to lose weight for the long term.

DIY low-calorie diet – If you opt-out of the Nutrisystem diet after a month this would be what you would be doing. The idea is to just fix small meal portions for yourself, be well informed with the calorie content of the foods you eat, and just make sure that you eat less than the normal daily allowance. The hard thing about this is that while it is cheaper you are left entirely alone to your devices. I was able to do this a few years ago but I stopped after a month because it was getting harder to constantly cook meals for myself and my motivation got lower the longer it went.

Conclusion

Go for the Nutrisystem diet. The convenience of having the food prepared for me in advance and have delicious meals available for me to choose just made it so much easier for me to lose weight. Having to prepare my snacks on weekdays and knowing what to eat and what not to eat on the weekends helped me develop a habit of taking care of myself. On the other hand not worrying about what to eat during my workdays continued to motivate me to lose weight. I have already ordered for the second month and I plan to do this for a few months more just so I can hit my weight target. After that, I think the habit of eating healthy will be well-ingrained in my mind that I will have no problem keeping off the weight I have lost. Now excuse me while I enjoy my last turkey sausage and egg muffin.

Made in the USA
Monee, IL
12 April 2021